Reactive Hypoglycemia

Reactive Hypoglycemia

✦

A Personal Journey Into Managing This Condition

K. E. LYTLE

iUniverse, Inc.

New York Lincoln Shanghai

Reactive Hypoglycemia
A Personal Journey Into Managing This Condition

Copyright © 2007 by K.E. Lytle

iUniverse books may be ordered through booksellers or by contacting:

iUniverse
2021 Pine Lake Road, Suite 100
Lincoln, NE 68512
www.iuniverse.com
1-800-Authors (1-800-288-4677)

Because of the dynamic nature of the Internet, any Web addresses or links contained in this book may have changed since publication and may no longer be valid.

ISBN: 978-0-595-47021-1 (pbk)
ISBN: 978-0-595-91305-3 (ebk)

Printed in the United States of America

Contents

ACKNOWLEDGMENTS

First and foremost, I would like to thank God for being there for me and leading me out of the darkness when I didn't know what was wrong.

I would like to dedicate this book to my brother who provided me with support, love, strength and concern through the whole ordeal. Thank you J for being my rock.

I would like to thank MW who responded when she didn't have to. She was the beacon of light in the darkness that led me to the answer. I will always be eternally grateful to her.

I would like to thank the Endocrinologist who gave me my life back. Even today, I want to cry when thinking of him. He was truly my hope when I had no hope.

And I want to thank all those who took time out of their lives to take me back and forth to the ER and to doctor's appointments and provided me with moral support. You know who you are. Thank you for your kindness.

Much love.

INTRODUCTION

INTRODUCTION

Being a private person, only a few people know that I have reactive hypoglycemia. When most people see the way I eat, they make the assumption that I'm just watching my weight or trying to be health conscious, so I just let them think that. I have found that it works better for me that way, as I do not have to try and explain to them why I shouldn't eat certain foods. And since I'm disciplined enough to stay away from the foods that are wrong for me, I can eat right along side people and no one is the wiser.

But, I wanted to write this book for people who have experienced, or are experiencing, reactive hypoglycemia, so that you can see that by sticking to certain food choices and eating at designated intervals throughout the day, you can keep your blood sugar stable and have a regular or even a great life, just like people who are able to eat whatever and whenever they want. By eating correctly, someone who has reactive hypoglycemia can eventually get to a point where they can have a small portion, and I do mean small, of the forbidden foods once in a while, without suffering severe effects.

So, my hope is that this book will inspire, educate, and motivate you in your quest for better health and for control of your reactive hypoglycemia.

When I was first told that I had reactive hypoglycemia, I read everything I could find on the subject. Although there were many good technical books on the subject, I rarely found any books that discussed it from a personal perspective. I longed to read the story of someone who had it and was living with it. I wanted to know what they went through on a daily basis. This is what inspired me to write this book. The book I wish I had to read when I didn't know how to control my reactive hypoglycemia. The book that I wanted to read before I got my health under control and was going through the debilitating, severe, symptoms of reactive hypoglycemia.

I hope that by reading my story, it reassures you that you can live a regular life if you are diligent about managing your condition. Those were the words I told the Endocrinologist when he explained to me that I had reactive hypoglycemia and would have to change the way I ate forever. I remember telling him that I just wanted to be a regular person, to eat like regular people do, and not feel sick. For a long time after I met with him, that's what bothered me the most. I just wanted to be able to eat like everybody else, whenever and whatever I wanted. I didn't want to restrict what I ate or adhere to a schedule of when to eat. I didn't want to have to be conscientious about what I was eating and what ingredients meals and foods had in them or whether it was a high glycemic or low glycemic food. Most people don't have to do that. "Regular people" just ate whatever they wanted to. But, as I soon learned, if I wanted to feel better, I was going to have to change the way I ate.

In the beginning, when I first began to have symptoms of reactive hypoglycemia, even the slightest variations of the sugar content of foods caused my blood sugar to fluctuate. I had to learn to be one hundred percent compliant with what and when I ate in order to achieve better health. I had to make sure that if I did happen to eat a food that caused a reaction, I was extremely compliant with the rest of the meals left for that particular day. I was, and continue to be, aware of how ill I can feel when I don't eat correctly and that the symptoms from eating incorrectly, simply lay dormant, always right there under the surface, waiting for me to make a mistake in what I eat, so they can spring to the surface once again.

Today, I enjoy the best of health and do not suffer from the severe symptoms of reactive hypoglycemia like I did in the beginning. This is because I have learned the hard way, what to eat and what not to eat, and I am disciplined about making certain food choices and eating at certain intervals throughout the day. I participate in many athletic activities including competing in 5K running events, 26 mile cycling events, and 10K inline skating events. I also ice skate, play tennis, swim, hike, and work out with weights. I am not in any way, removed from living life because of reactive hypoglycemia. I simply have to make sure to eat correctly and to eat at certain intervals.

That is the main thing about having this condition that I want to emphasis, that you can never "forget" or "pretend" that you don't have it. Because if you do, your body is right there to remind you. Oh, you can mask your symptoms to the world around you, by just saying that you have a headache or don't feel well or something, so that others won't know that you have a "condition", but *you* will know that the real reason you are not feeling well is because you ate something you shouldn't have. And in the end, you are the one who will be harmed. It is your body that is harmed. So, it is my hope that this book will show you that you can take control over this condition and not let it take control over you.

Some people mistakenly believe that the condition hypoglycemia, which literally means low blood sugar, is the opposite of diabetes or hyperglycemia, which literally means high blood sugar. However, in fact, reactive hypoglycemia is often thought by many medical professionals to be a pre-diabetic state which sometimes precede one developing diabetes mellitus type II, but not always. Many professionals believe that reactive hypoglycemia is due to insulin resistance, or the cells in the body becoming resistant to the effects of insulin. This resistance causes the pancreas to secrete large amounts of insulin in response to fast absorbing carbohydrates such as sugars and refined carbohydrates. It is believed that all diabetics with diabetes mellitus, type II, have insulin resistance and that those people with reactive hypoglycemia have just not gotten to the point yet where enough of their cells are resistant to cause diabetes. In reactive hypoglycemia, although some of the cells may be *becoming* insulin resistant, they have not yet begun to stop accepting the sugar carried in by the insulin. As such, some people who develop reactive hypoglycemia, simply have reactive hypoglycemia the rest of their lives and never develop diabetes mellitus, type II. Others, however, who do not change their diet and increase exercise, or simply because of genetics, may eventually go on to develop diabetes mellitus, type II. Other factors such as family history, increasing age, race, weight, and lifestyle also contribute to developing diabetes.

What is reactive hypoglycemia? Reactive hypoglycemia occurs when someone has a "reaction" to eating certain types of food. Foods that contain various sugars or simple carbohydrates such as white rice, white flour, pasta, various breads, potatoes, etc., cause the blood sugar to drop too fast and/or too low in people with reactive hypoglycemia. In response to eating these foods, instead of the body releasing the correct amount of insulin, the pancreas *overreacts* and releases an abundance of insulin, which in turn floods the bloodstream with too much insulin, which then causes the insulin to remove too much sugar from the bloodstream or to remove the sugar too quickly from the bloodstream, thereby causing symptoms from the lack of adequate blood sugar for the body to function properly. This can occur soon after eating or a couple of hours after eating, depending on how fast the pancreas overreacts. When there is not enough sugar in the blood for the body to function properly, symptoms will occur. Since the brain and nervous system use sugar or glucose for fuel, many of the symptoms experienced are related to a deficiency of sugar or glucose being felt in these two body systems.

Additionally, the body is equipped with an emergency system that responds when the blood sugar falls too low or too quickly. The adrenal glands release adrenalin, which tells the liver to release glycogen to raise the blood sugar level. The liver contains a small storage of glucose for emergencies called glycogen. However, when this adrenalin is released to raise the blood sugar, a person will experience an *additional host of symptoms due to the effects of the adrenalin,* which not only serves to raise the blood glucose level by activating the liver to release glycogen, but also to raise blood pressure as well. Often, the adrenal glands, like the pancreas, will be over-reactive as well in someone with reactive hypoglycemia. Therefore, someone experiencing reactive hypoglycemia, can become totally non-functional from the host of symptoms that occur from the actual low sugar level in the blood and from the effects of an abundance of adrenalin in the system.

Below are some of the many symptoms of reactive hypoglycemia. Someone with a severe case, can experience all these symptoms at one time from a reaction to certain foods:

- shaking

- trembling

- sweating

- convulsions

- fainting and/or blackouts

- unresponsiveness

- sudden sleepiness

- numbness

- muscle weakness

- irritability for no reason

- confusion and altered mental status

- repetitive unclear speech

- inability to speak

- blurred vision

- fast heart rate

- lightheadedness

- dizziness

- tingling

- headache

- inability to sleep

- nausea

- extreme hunger

- coma

These symptoms are the result of the brain and nervous system not having enough glucose to operate properly and from the adrenalin that is released when the body experiences a low blood sugar attack.

As you can see, it can be quite debilitating and scary. In a severe attack, when one is experiencing the majority of these symptoms at the same time, a person can become totally non-functional. The symptoms are the exact same symptoms diabetics have when their blood sugar levels become too low. The only treatment during an attack is to bring the body's blood sugar level back to a normal state by eating or drinking something that will cause the sugar level to rise and remain stable.

It is important to remember that a low blood sugar attack due to reactive hypoglycemia can be brought on not just by the low sugar level itself, but also by how fast the blood sugar level drops or descends after eating certain foods. In the beginning, when I was having severe reactive hypoglycemia and didn't know that I had it, I would eat something I now know I shouldn't eat, and within twenty to thirty minutes, I would feel a dropping sensation in my head like I was going to faint. I often had to grab hold of something, because everything would go black and I felt like I was going to pass out. At the time, it scared me because I didn't know what was happening and I thought I was about to drop dead or something. I would also get really sweaty, often to the point that I was literally dripping with sweat. My hands, and even my face, would get shaky and my heart would beat really fast. My arms or legs would sometimes go numb and my eyesight would become blurry. I wouldn't be able to think clearly and would feel confused. All I could do was suffer. If you have ever seen a diabetic experience a low blood sugar attack or hypoglycemia, the symptoms are the same that occurs in reactive hypoglycemia.

I hope that by telling you my story, no one will have to suffer to the degree that I did and for those that are, that this book will show you that you don't have to.

1

IN THE BEGINNING

IN THE BEGINNING

It all started around May 2002. I began experiencing strange symptoms, that got progressively worse. Actually, I had been experiencing some of the same symptoms a couple of months earlier, just on a milder level.

In May 2002, I participated in a 5K running event. After the race, there were refreshments that the events routinely give away to participants. The refreshment box consisted of fast acting carbohydrates including juices, raisins, snack bars, bagels, and candy bars. I remember feeling kind of lightheaded at the time, so I ate two refreshment boxes. For the rest of the day and days following, I didn't feel well. I constantly felt lightheaded and faint, sweaty, rapid heart rate, disoriented, sleepy, shaky, trembling, and numbness in my extremities. Looking back, I now know that eating all that sugar in those refreshment boxes only made things worse because all the excessive insulin that was released just further lowered my blood sugar and did nothing to replenish the glycogen stores that we have in our liver.

As days went on, there would be times while I was sitting at my desk at work when my legs or arms would suddenly go numb. My legs would feel like dead weight, like I had lead for legs. I would also sometimes have severe nerve pain, where I would feel a burning pain traveling the length of my arms or legs. My eyes would sometimes burn as well. This numbness and nerve pain would come and go or sometimes last for a couple of days. During these episodes, I would also get really hot and sweaty, my heart would beat extremely fast, my eyes would get blurry, and I would feel lightheaded and confused. I often felt like I was going to faint and fall right out of my chair. I would also get really shaky, sometimes so bad that I thought I must be having a seizure, but yet I was conscious. These episodes would come on any time of the day and also during the night, and initially, seemed to be random as to when they would occur.

Over time, it seemed like the episodes became more frequent and more intense. I even began to have the episodes while driving in my car and I often felt so faint that I thought I would end up crashing my car into someone. Finally, they became so bad, I could no longer make it to work, let alone work once I was able to get there. I ended up having to take three weeks of sick leave from my job, which was the most leave I had ever taken off in my life from a job. Up until that point, I had never taken more than three consecutive days off from work due to illness, let alone three weeks. During my three weeks off work, I was so extremely sick with these episodes that I was barely able to get out of bed. And even just laying in bed, the episodes would continue.

I went in to see the doctor and underwent a battery of tests, including x-rays, urine tests, blood tests, CAT scans, MRI's of the brain, and a neurological exam. I was given B-12 injections, epilepsy medication, migraine medication, and anxiety medication. Nothing helped.

That experience made me recall how approximately a year earlier, I was having some bad stomach problems. At that time, I was nauseated and bloated every day. It was constant and severe. I tried practically every kind of over the counter stomach medication on the market, to no avail. That went on for about a year before I got up the courage to go to the doctor. They thought that maybe I didn't have enough enzymes to digest my food and gave me enzyme tablets to try, which did not work. I kept telling them over and over that it seemed like my food was not digesting, but just sitting in my stomach and intestines and fermenting. They just thought I was crazy. They gave me a battery of tests including a barium x-ray, an endoscopy, and a colonoscopy. The barium x-ray consisted of eating a peanut butter and jelly sandwich on white bread while you lay under this machine for two hours as it tracks how long the food stays in your stomach. Based on that test, they told me that I had idiopathic gastroparesis and prescribed medication for that, which didn't help at all. Next, they told me I had h-pylori, which is a bacteria infection that can affect the digestive system. They prescribed two types of antibiotics and some kind of acid inhibitor for me to take for ten days. It was horrendous and made me feel sick as a dog. Afterwards, I initially felt better for a few days, but to this day, I now realize that when I eat an abundance of carbohydrates, I get those same stomach symptoms, along with symptoms of reactive hypoglycemia.

Anyway, during my three weeks off, as one week turned into another, and doctors couldn't tell me what was wrong and with my job becoming concerned about when I was coming back to work, I became desperate for some relief from the unbearable symptoms and to find out what was wrong with me. So, I decided to go out on a limb and pay out of pocket to go see a doctor outside the care system I was in at the time. I felt like I was suffering and was willing to pay any amount to find out what was wrong. I felt like I had no choice. I was too sick to go back to work, but yet I needed to. I couldn't just lose my job and become unemployed. I had started a career and wanted and needed to work. And I couldn't just lay there in bed suffering all day and night with no relief. I had become non-functional. I was constantly lightheaded and not able to concentrate. My limbs were shaky, my heart was constantly beating uncontrollably fast, and I had numbness in either my legs or arms or both. I didn't know where to start so I thought that maybe it was my heart that was causing all the problems. Maybe I had developed a heart condition. So I made an appointment with a cardiologist. The cardiologist did an extensive EKG and didn't find anything wrong with my heart. I was happy about that, but now I was back to wondering what could be wrong with me.

During those three weeks off from work, I was often so sick with the symptoms, that I had to have various people drive me to the ER several times. One time that I had to go to the ER occurred after I had taken a nap and woke up shaking so bad, that looking back now, I do believe that I had a convulsion. It was very frightening. My limbs seemed to be out of my control and shaking involuntarily. I also felt like I had swelling in my head. When I went to the ER, they just said they didn't know what was wrong and referred me to see a Neurologist, after giving me an x-ray and epilepsy medication. I became desperate to find some relief. I researched in medical books and on the internet. For some reason, I thought maybe I should try drinking some salt water because maybe my blood pressure was falling too low. I thought that maybe that was the problem. So, I forced myself to drink as many glasses of salt water as I could. Needless to say, this did not help me at all and only made things worse, as my feet swelled up like balloons. I then became scared that I had now thrown off my electrolyte balance by drinking all that salt water and thought that now something else was going to happen to me. I then tried to drink as much water as I could to help clear the salt out of my body. I eventually had to go back to the ER and told them what I had done.

I then returned to searching the internet when I felt physically able to do so. As days went on, I began to notice that the symptoms did not seem to just come on randomly like I had initially thought. I began to notice that the symptoms were coming on in a pattern, within about a half hour to an hour after I finished eating. That then made me think that maybe I had developed some kind of severe allergy to certain foods. That I had suddenly became allergic to certain foods and that I was having a severe allergic attack of some kind. I then began to research food allergies. My research showed me that to find out what food allergies one has, one should go on a non-allergic diet consisting of white rice and lamb. Then after eating only white rice and lamb for a while, gradually add back different foods to see if you react to any of them. So, that's what I did. After several days of eating nothing but white rice and lamb for every meal of the day, including breakfast, there was no change, and my episodes continued.

So, I went back to the internet. Then, by the grace of God, I came across a Web site that described the exact symptoms I was experiencing. Every single symptom I was experiencing, was listed on this Web site. The Web site was on reactive hypoglycemia. It talked about how sugary foods, and refined carbohydrates, caused the blood sugar to drop in people who had this condition. It described how after eating sugar or refined carbohydrates, the pancreas secretes too much insulin in response to these foods. This particular Web site explained how some people, because of a family history of diabetes, genetics, and/or years of eating this type of diet, will develop reactive hypoglycemia and have a hyper insulin response, due to cell damage or insulin resistance. The Web site indicated that the woman who had developed the site, also had reactive hypoglycemia, and at that time, was 66 years old. The Web site also contained her e-mail address. So, I decided to email her. At that time, I had never e-mailed anyone I didn't know, but because I was so severely sick and desperate for help, I was willing to take a chance. I didn't think she would e-mail me back and that even if she did, that it would probably take several days or even weeks before she responded. But, again, by the grace of God, she responded the very next day! I told her my situation and informed her what state and city I lived in. On her Web site, she had stated that she lived in another state on the east coast. She informed me of an excellent Endocrinologist at one of the most prestigious medical centers in Los Angeles. I was thrilled. I just felt hopeful that maybe, just maybe, this doctor could help me. She gave me his name and e-mail address and I e-mailed him right away.

However, my hopes were soon dashed when someone from his staff called and told me that he was booked up for the next six months or so. I begged to be seen and told them I would pay any cost. I told them that cost didn't matter, I had to see him. Finally, after what I thought was going to be hopeless, they were able to squeeze me in. In the meantime, I called my regular doctor and made a same day appointment and insisted that I wanted to take a blood sugar test. They scheduled me for the test and I went in and was given a sugary drink to drink and was told to sit in the waiting room for two hours. At the end of the two hours, they took my blood sugar. It was 71. A normal blood sugar is approximately 85-100. Anything around a 75, 70, 65, and certainly below this, can cause symptoms. (I have since bought a blood sugar monitor and have had several readings in the 50's and 60's during a severe episode). Anyway, when I saw my regular doctor, who was a general practitioner, and not a specialist in the field of Endocrinology, he just made a comment that my blood sugar was on the low side and that it was better to have a lower sugar reading, than a high sugar reading, because a high reading would mean I was diabetic. While I was glad that I was not diabetic, the point not mentioned was that while a diabetic can have a blood sugar reading that is 30-50mg or even higher *above the normal level* and not feel any noticeable difference at all, someone who has a *drop* of blood sugar of 30-50mg *below the normal level*, will most definitely feel ill and have symptoms, because the brain and nervous system cannot function with a low supply of sugar in the blood, as glucose is the only source of fuel for these body systems. Which is why too low of sugar in the blood will cause immediate symptoms, whereas too high of sugar in the blood usually does not, unless of course, it is extremely high.

Anyway, my primary doctor just told me to try and eat more frequently. That was it. That was the extent of the discussion.

After I left, I immediately went to patient records to request all my medical records so that I could take them with me when I saw the Endocrinologist. When I finally had my appointment with the Endocrinologist, I immediately liked him. He was very patient and very kind. He interviewed me, examined me, and reviewed my medical records. He looked at my blood sugar test and told me that as a specialist in Endocrinology, he had seen many patients over the years and had written many books as well as given lectures on all kinds of endocrine problems. He told me that he was not going to put me through any more tests because based on his medical opinion and experience, I had reactive hypoglycemia. He then explained to me what it was, and what happens in the body of someone who has it. He told me that based on my family history, it was likely I was developing a pre-diabetic condition. He even drew a diagram for me to keep, which showed what happens when the pancreas overreacts. He gave me a food list designed for those with reactive hypoglycemia, which identified what foods to avoid and which foods were okay to eat. He also instructed me to eat every two and a half or three hours and not to exercise for a couple of months until my blood sugar had become more stable. He also told me that people with reactive hypoglycemia often get a lot of bloating and nausea when they eat large amounts of carbohydrates as their bodies are not able to effectively utilize an abundance of carbohydrates, which can often sit in the intestines undigested. I was so grateful to him, it was like God had led me to him. I gave him a hug when I left and was so happy that when I got in my car, I just sat there and cried. Finally, I knew what was wrong and could begin to get better.

I immediately began following the food restriction list and within a matter of days, I began to feel much better. I felt it was truly a miracle. I still had the episodes, they were not totally gone that fast, but within days, the episodes were less intense. However, after about two weeks of following the food restriction list, the episodes had not completely disappeared, so I decided to make a follow-up appointment to see the Endocrinologist again. He informed me that because my pancreas had gone for a long period of time in an overactive state, that it was going to take awhile for it to realize that it did not have to over-react to everything I ate anymore. He informed me that my pancreas was still over-secreting insulin because my cells were becoming resistant to insulin (or insulin resistant). He indicated that to give my pancreas a chance to rest, he wanted me to take a diabetes medication that would help alleviate insulin resistance. So, I started taking it and I noticed a difference within the first few days. I had a lot more energy and just felt great. The episodes lessened and I was thrilled. But, after about a month of taking it, my feet started to swell, so I discontinued it.

I continued on with the food restriction and as I began to feel better, I included some exercise into my routine, which at first was a real challenge. Exercise lowers the blood sugar, for everyone, which is why they tell diabetics, who have high blood sugar, to exercise. If you have reactive hypoglycemia, your body is already causing you to have low blood sugar, so you have to be especially careful that the exercise doesn't further lower an already low blood sugar. By sticking to the restricted diet, you are able to maintain a *normal* blood sugar level, versus constantly having a low blood sugar level. This normal blood sugar level will allow you to be able to exercise without having any severe effects. However, as mentioned, since exercise does lower the blood sugar, people with reactive hypoglycemia must make sure to eat after engaging in strenuous exercise to counteract the sugar lowering effects of the exercise. It is also wise not to exercise on an empty stomach since your sugar level is already low if you haven't eaten and will just go lower after exercise. Also, since the sugar lowering effects of exercise can carry over into the next day, it is very important to be disciplined in sticking to the restricted diet and eating intervals.

The endocrinologist informed me to eat at least five to six times a day, every two and a half to three hours, versus just eating one or two large meals a day. The five or six meals did not have to be large meals and in fact, should not be overly large portions of food. But the meals should be enough food to carry you to the next meal and must always include some protein and a little fat and fiber, as fat and fiber slows down the digestion process and prevents spikes in your blood sugar. In the beginning, when I had severe symptoms, I had to eat a snack every night before bedtime, otherwise I would wake up in the night with an episode, since night time is a long span of time to go without eating. But over time, as my body began to stabilize, I now no longer have to have a bedtime snack, as long as I eat a substantial meal for dinner. Additionally, before my blood sugar became stable, I would often wake in the morning feeling shaky with an episode coming on, but again, since changing my eating style, I no longer have this problem.

Although within a matter of months, I was able to become a functional person again, it really took close to a year to feel totally great, at one hundred percent. This is because I had to learn how I reacted to different foods. During this year, I learned a lot about foods, carbohydrates, the different types of carbohydrates, the glycemic index, fiber, fats, and how they all react in the body. Something the average person probably never thinks about. I learned that for me, in the beginning, a regular serving of fruit could be intolerable. Some people with this condition are able to tolerate fruit as long as it is eaten with some protein. But for me, fruit, or more specifically, the natural sugar in fruit, fructose, is one of my worst offenders. I tried every kind of fruit in the grocery markets. I tried half pieces of fruit. I tried fruit that was considered low glycemic. I ate fruit with various types of protein. But, no matter how I tried it, fruit always bothered me. So, I totally gave up fruit for a while and I felt one hundred percent better for having done so. It really made a big difference. Now, however, I am able to tolerate very small portions of fruit eaten periodically, and always with some protein, never by itself.

I also learned that I felt better when I ate my whole grains in the morning versus in the evening hours. So, for the most part, I try not to eat grains in the evening. I also seem to have a total carbohydrate limit that when I go over, seems to cause problems. For example, I can have a bowl of steel cut oatmeal or whole grain cereal with soymilk and almonds for breakfast and be fine. Because it is whole grains and not refined flour, it will not cause a reaction. Plus, the soymilk and almonds provide protein and fiber which slows absorption. But if were to eat two or three bowls of this at one sitting, even though one bowl would not cause a reaction, eating two or three bowls *would* cause a reaction. So, just because a food is considered okay for a reactive hypoglycemic to eat, doesn't mean that you can gorge on that food and not have any problems.

I also found that if I eat a food that I shouldn't eat, it not only throws my system off for that day, but can have a carry over effect into the next day or two, before my body is once again, back to a stabilized position. For that reason, if I eat something I shouldn't, I try to be extra diligent the rest of the day and the next day, to lessen the negative effects. The pancreas seems to want to revert back to its over-reactive state and only by adhering to the food restrictions and eating intervals, does it get back on the right track. For me, that has showed me that no matter how great I feel, I know that the reactive hypoglycemia is not "cured" or gone away, and is always right there under the surface, waiting to revert back. And after what I went through, the memory alone is enough to keep me in line. And if the memory of what I went through isn't enough, the symptoms, even if minor now, are enough to refresh my memory of how severe it can be if I don't eat correctly.

It took a while for me to learn that lesson. Many times, months would go by and I would feel one hundred percent, just great. I felt like I was "back to normal". That I no longer had reactive hypoglycemia. I would forget that I felt great **because** I had been in strict compliance with what I ate. And so, I would mistakenly think that now I could eat a bag of cookies again, because I must be "cured" since I felt so great. And then I would be brought back to reality. All the symptoms would start again. That was one of the hardest lessons I had to learn. That I couldn't go back to those bad eating habits. And for a long time, I was filled with self pity. I felt sorry for myself because I couldn't just eat a box of donuts if I wanted to. I had hoped that one day I would be able to eat like that again, like I used to. I thought that since I felt great, I could resume eating all the things I used to be able to eat. But, I finally learned, that not only is that unhealthy for everybody, it just makes me ill from reactive hypoglycemia. And I like feeling well way more than feeling good for the five minutes it takes to polish off a bag of cookies and then having to pay the price for it by being sick later. So for me, having the discipline to eat correctly, is no problem whatsoever.

Additionally, I continue to stay educated in both reactive hypoglycemia and diabetes and hope that by doing so, along with my healthy diet and exercise regimen, that I can prevent myself from developing diabetes mellitus, type II in the future.

Although genetics and family history are strong factors in the development of type II diabetes, lifestyle choices also play a major role in the prevention and subsequent development of this condition. If nothing else, it can give you better health and vitality in your day to day life.

NOTES

2

FAMILY HISTORY

FAMILY HISTORY

As a child and young adult, I was like everyone else, I ate anything, at anytime. Food was in abundance, as it seems to be in the United States. However, like most kids, I loved sugary foods and often stuffed myself with as much ice cream, candy, donuts, cupcakes, pudding, cakes, and pie as I wanted. And, when I think back to those days, I have many fond memories. It was great. I simply loved sugary foods. I enjoyed every minute of everything I ate. I remember stopping by the bakery on the way home from school. They had everything. It was a magical delight of pastries. I can still visualize that bakery today. The apple pies were especially delicious. But, everything was yummy. And I ate as much as my money could buy.

I have fond memories of looking forward to the ice cream truck coming around the neighborhood every evening. In the summertime, it would often come by twice a day. I remember there was a smaller truck that came by and also a larger pink and white striped truck that would come by. We called the pink and white striped truck, "the big ice cream truck", because it had everything. Popsicles, a variety of ice cream, banana splits, everything. There were some I can still visualize today but don't remember the names. I loved all of them. And of course, I drank soda like there was no tomorrow. Never even heard of *diet* soda in those days. I drank gallons of soda, punch, and juices all day long.

Then there were the times when a group of friends would get together and walk to the store and buy snacks. I would never just have one, but two or three of whatever I would buy. And of course, we always bought some candy to eat for later. And maybe some chips too.

In my junior high school, as well as in high school, for break time or nutrition time as they called it then, which was usually around 9-10:00 am, I would often go to the little student store we had on campus that sold candy. And that is what I would eat for my break. Every single day, it was candy. I would often eat candy for lunch as well. Candy and nothing else. Sometimes, in addition to candy, I would have what they called coffee cakes, which was some kind of cinnamon muffin that the cafeteria would sell hot. And then there were other times when I would just have a bag of chips and a hotdog or something like that.

And then of course, like most kids, I ate at all the fast food restaurants, eating my share of burgers, fries, pizza, burritos, tacos, malts, etc.

Then there were the times when my mom would take us out for breakfast on Sunday morning after church. That was great too. I would order a big stack of pancakes and drown them in maple syrup. Or sometimes I would get waffles with straw-berry syrup and whip cream on top.

Oh, those were the days. Although I no longer crave those sugary delights, just thinking about them makes me wish I could eat like that again. With total abandon. I have such happy emotions tied to eating those foods and being able to eat anything I wanted to without worry of the consequences. They always made me feel good by how they tasted. The joy of childhood.

I never had a weight problem, maybe because my mother was naturally thin all her life. Or maybe because in my younger years, I also loved sports and athletics, and even though I gorged on sugary foods, I also got a high amount of exercise every day.

As I got older though, into my late twenties, I found that sug-ary foods seemed to make me feel kind of funny. Juices and tomato sauces did as well. I would feel kind of lightheaded if I ate or drank too much of these foods. I would also get a little jittery and get a headache when I didn't eat. Nothing at all compared to now. But just enough to notice that I would not feel so great after gorging on these foods. I just assumed that everybody felt the same way, so I really didn't think much about it. I actually remember asking people if they felt shaky when they skipped meals. Most people would just say no, so I never gave it any further thought. At that time, it was no big deal, as I would just eat something, anything, and I would feel much better. I do recall though, that when I was in my late twenties, there was a lady that I worked with, who was about thirty years older than I was, who said to me one day as we were driving on a business trip, that we were going to have to pull over and get some lunch because she got shaky when she didn't eat. I remember thinking at the time that I got that way too. But while I can look back now and say that those were hypoglycemic symptoms, low blood sugar, it was mild in comparison to what I experienced years later. But, as in many conditions, one doesn't just go to bed perfectly fine, and wake up the next day, in a severe state. Often, things gradually get worse over time, unless you intervene and do something about it.

In diabetes mellitus, type II, a lot of people go through a pre-diabetes or borderline diabetes stage, before they become full fledged diabetic. During this stage, with proper diet and exercise, many people can prevent developing diabetes or delay it for many, many years. As such, many people are lucky to have a wake-up call to make changes to prevent diabetes from occurring. Others, do not make changes, and as the pancreas becomes more and more worn down from being overactive, combined with the genetics of that particular individual, it may no longer be able to function effectively and one will become diabetic. That is why I have to say that I consider being reactive hypoglycemic the best thing to happen to me, health-wise. I say this because I know that if I didn't have this condition, I would still be gorging on sugary foods to the same degree that I did as a child. I would have no reason not to. The only other deterrent that would probably prevent me from eating that way would be if I started to put on weight, but as long as I remained thin, I know that I would still be eating that way, which I know now, is totally unhealthy.

When I was growing up, my mom told me that my father, had "sugar". That's how she phrased it, "you know your dad had "sugar". My father passed away when I was four, unrelated to diabetes. My mom also said to me that one time the doctor told my father that if he didn't change his diet, they were going to have to put him on pills to control his sugar. That's all I knew about my father's condition, which of course we know today that "sugar" meant diabetes. Later, in my twenties, I learned that my father's mother, my grandmother, also had diabetes. She had to go on dialysis and was almost blind. She lived on the east coast so I never knew many details of her diabetes. When my brother graduated from college, my grandmother came to the graduation and she could barely walk. She was very ill and her eyes were watery and cloudy. But again, no one really talked to me about the exact nature of her condition. All I was told was that she had diabetes, and was on dialysis, that was it. Later, in my thirties, I learned from a cousin, that my father's brother had diabetes as well, and had both of his legs amputated. Again, I do not know what other secondary complications he experienced. This same cousin told me that she also got shaky, jittery, sweats, lightheaded, etc., when she didn't eat or after eating sugary or refined carbohydrates. The same as me. My great grandmother, the mother of my father's mother, had a wooden leg, but I do not know if she had diabetes or not. All I know is that as a child, I saw her with a wooden leg.

When you have relatives that are located all over the country, it is often hard to find out exactly who has what kind of illnesses in your family line. Also, often times, family members, for whatever reason, just do not want to share the details of conditions of other family members. But, knowing your family's medical history is very important, especially in conditions that have a genetic or hereditary base, such as with diabetes mellitus, type II.

I often think that if I had been aware of my full family history, had been counseled by medical professionals to not over indulge in certain foods since I have a genetic predisposition for developing diabetes, maybe I wouldn't have gorged myself on sugary foods throughout my life. And maybe I wouldn't have reactive hypoglycemia today.

But since you can't go back in time, I can only hope that with all that I have learned about reactive hypoglycemia and diabetes, that by following good eating patterns now and continuing to engage in exercise, that I will avoid getting diabetes and continue to be healthy.

NOTES

3

WORK AND SOCIAL LIFE

WORK AND SOCIAL LIFE

One of the hardest adjustments I had with reactive hypoglycemia and changing my eating style, was not so much with
myself, but in dealing with other people. Since most adults
continue to eat the way I did as a child, a lot of people find it
strange when they see the way I eat now. I have found that
most people will freely comment on what you are eating or the
fact that you are eating "again". And since I keep my private
life to myself, most people just assume I eat the way I do
because I am trying to stay slim. Still, others have made com-
ments that I must be trying to live "forever" because I eat so
healthy all the time. I guess since most people tend to just eat
whatever and whenever they feel like it, when they see someone who isn't eating like them, they think it's strange. I've also
noticed that a lot of people have erratic eating schedules. If,
for example, they want to eat lunch at 11:00 a.m. today, they
do so. If they then don't want to eat anything else until late
evening, say for example, until around 8:00 p.m., they do so.
If they feel like having a snack an hour after that, they eat one.
The next day, they might change up and eat lunch at 1:30
p.m. if they felt like it, or just skip lunch altogether. Other
people wake up in the morning and don't eat a bite until 1:00
or 2:00 in the afternoon. Still, others may have a donut first
thing in the morning. Or, just snack on junk food all day
long. I have found it fascinating to see the eating styles of
other people, I guess the same way they find the way I eat fas-

cinating. I guess it just amazes me because it is so very different than the way I eat now and I know that I would feel ill if I ate their way.

In my work life, I have also made the choice to not tell anyone that the reason why I eat the way I do is because of reactive hypoglycemia. I just do not want to be asked a thousand questions. It took a lot of explaining and educating the few people that I have told in my personal life, and I just don't want to deal with it in the workplace. Also, I do not want people thinking I am different in some way, because to me, it is just a condition that requires that I eat differently, it is not who I am. So, when we have parties at work or someone brings in a box of donuts, or when we have a potluck, and coworkers see me either not participating or being selective in what I eat, I just tell them that I am trying to watch my figure and let it go as that. Since I've done that for so long, everyone just believes I am weight conscious. Which is fine by me.

The only problem I have with this approach is that some coworkers will continue to pressure me by telling me that it would be okay for me to have "one slice of pizza, or one small donut". Some people get personally offended when you don't join in and indulge like they are doing. Since I am thin, a lot of people think that there is no reason why I shouldn't "pig out" once in a while. Most people don't even think or care that the food itself is unhealthy for *anybody*, not just for those with certain medical conditions.

In addition, another thing I have found in interacting with people, both personally and professionally, is that I know of several diabetics who freely partake of sugary foods at various get togethers or parties, and don't think twice about it. Some of these same people have even prodded me to partake in these sugary foods, when they shouldn't be eating it themselves! But, it is like I mentioned earlier, a diabetic can experience a rise in blood sugar and often not feel any differently, but someone with reactive hypoglycemia cannot tolerate a *drop* in blood sugar without often feeling immediate symptoms. Therefore, it is more imperative that reactive hypoglycemics try to stick to the eating restrictions at all times.

The other work issue I find challenging is trying to eat when it is time for me to eat. Often there is some emergency, some issue, some unforeseen event, where someone needs me to do something right at the time that I should eat. Or, I am busy trying to finish up on something that I am working on to stop and eat. So to alleviate eating too late, I will often try to eat a half hour earlier than my normal time, which I have found works out fine. Other times, delays cannot be avoided, so I will just either eat while I am working or as soon as the event is over, and then just adjust my schedule for the remainder of the day.

If your blood sugar is not stable and you are experiencing severe symptoms, everyday can be a challenge. When you are involved with work, social activities, and just everyday life, trying to juggle all of that, and also trying to eat correctly, can sometimes be overwhelming. A lot of people are not understanding because they have never experienced a low blood sugar attack. They don't know what it's like to almost pass out because your blood sugar is too low. Having people in your life who are understanding and not judgmental, are invaluable. In the beginning, I received a lot of support from an online support group devoted to those with reactive hypoglycemia. The people on this support group were wonderful. I also chatted with people on several online diabetic support groups, as many of them experience hypoglycemic episodes because of the medication or insulin they take, or because they first had reactive hypoglycemia before they became diabetic. Although I no longer have a need to frequent these groups, I have learned a lot from talking with other people and have gotten advice and ideas on how to manage this condition and how to prevent from becoming a diabetic in the future.

NOTES

4

MEALS

MEALS

When I was first told I had reactive hypoglycemia, the Endocrinologist gave me a food list containing food restrictions of what to eat and what not to eat. Basically, I was to eliminate all forms of sugar including honey, and all refined carbohydrates and high glycemic carbohydrates. I was to eliminate all refined grains or flour, including white bread, pasta, white rice, potatoes, as well as fruit juices, and foods and sauces containing sugar in them, as they are considered high glycemic foods, and turn into sugar quickly in the body. And I was to eat five or six meals a day, in two and a half to three hour intervals. Following the food list helped me tremendously. I did not deviate from it whatsoever. I was thrilled to feel so much better and really had no desire at all to eat anything off the list because I knew how sick it would make me feel. (Pain is a very strong deterrent).

To this day, I continue to follow the food list with a few other restrictions I had to add. As mentioned earlier, I cannot tolerate much fruit at all, so I only eat small portions of it. I also cannot tolerate any dairy products because of the milk sugar, lactose. My doctor told me to watch for hidden sugars on packages such as anything ending in "ose", like fructose. Additionally, there are many other forms of sugar that don't end in "ose" that you must also watch out for, that may or may not bother you, depending on your sensitivity level. For example, I cannot tolerate food items that contain fruit juice, yogurt, apple cider vinegar, sugar alcohols, or various sugar substitutes. I have also found that a lot of food products labeled as diabetic often are not good food choices for those with reactive hypoglycemia, depending upon your sensitivity. So, take caution with food items labeled as "sugar free". Please take note that through trial and error, I have found that the below food choices work best for me as I seem to be extra sensitive to sugar of any kind. Some people who are not as sensitive may be able to tolerate other food choices such as certain pastas or various cereals, or greater portion sizes of the same choices, such as fruit. I have experienced the worst, in reaction to consuming the wrong foods, so I tend to stick with what I know works best for me. The following is my typical meal schedule:

Breakfast: 6am

Morning Snack: 9am

Lunch: 12 noon

Afternoon Snack: 3pm

Dinner: 6-7pm

Although I try to adhere to the same eating schedule everyday, often there are some variations due to unforeseen events. It is usually easier to adhere to this schedule Monday through Friday, as I have work to shape the day. On the weekends, when my schedule is more flexible, this schedule may vary from what is listed. I will try to eat every few hours though, they just may not occur at the time intervals listed. Since my life on Saturday and Sunday does not require a set time to be anywhere, I can't predict if I will be home or near a place to eat at any given time. Therefore, I just make sure to bring something to snack with me or leave some nuts in the car.

Breakfast:

I tend to rotate three different meals which consist of the following:

- Cold cereal. I have found only one cereal that I can eat that is made of whole grains and doesn't cause me symptoms. I have read of others recommended in some books as being low glycemic cereals, but I've tried them all, and for me, they all cause symptoms. So, I eat Ezekiel 4:9 cereal, which is made of whole grains and no sugar. I top it with almond slithers, flax seeds, and unsweetened soy milk. (This cereal comes with flaxseed and almonds, but I like to add more). I also add a few berries.

Or,

- Hot cereal. Steel cut oats is the only hot cereal I can eat that doesn't cause symptoms. It takes a long time to cook because it is whole grain. I also top it with almonds, sometimes a little cinnamon, and unsweetened soymilk. (I thought I would have to give up oatmeal because in the beginning, oatmeal was one of the main foods I had been eating for breakfast that caused severe symptoms. But, back then, I was eating the fast cook oatmeal, which is refined and not the whole grain, and can thus cause the blood sugar to spike in many people with reactive hypoglycemia).

Or,

- Eggs, turkey sausage or turkey bacon, with tomato slices or salsa, avocado slices, and one slice of Ezekiel bread. (When I eat this particular meal, it seems to stay with me longer).

Morning Snack:

To make life easier, I usually rotate two different morning snacks. These two snacks seem to stick with me enough to carry me to lunchtime:

- Sugar free peanut butter sandwich using Ezekiel bread. (Ezekiel bread is the only bread I have found that I can tolerate and I have tried all brands).

- Turkey sausage or turkey bacon sandwich with a slice of avocado and tomato using Ezekiel bread. (Sometimes I will just have a half of sandwich).

- After that, I usually eat no more grains for the day. That's my limit. Also, I will usually have a cup of hot green tea or herb tea with my morning snack.

Lunch:

Lunch always consist of the same food groups: some kind of meat and vegetables, and sometimes various types of beans. Period. I never eat any rice, potatoes, pasta, bread, etc. I typically have any of the following or some variation:

- Turkey burger with salsa and avocado on top or with soy cheese and a tomato slice on top, or with hummus, and a salad or some cooked mixed vegetables.

- Salmon, halibut, or some other fish with a salad or mixed vegetables.

- Home made stir fry consisting of turkey or chicken strips with stir fry mixed vegetables and maybe a little tofu

- Chicken breast or a turkey fillet with either a salad or mixed vegetables

- Home made chicken stew without pasta or tomato sauce. If I want some tomatoes in it, I will just chop up a few fresh tomatoes or use salsa.

- Chicken kebabs with a salad

- Home made ground turkey chili with beans and salsa

- Stuffed bell peppers

- Fajitas with beans, salsa, and guacamole

For my salads, I have found two salad dressings that do not use sugar in them. If I want some kind of sauce on my meat, I will use hot sauce or salsa, which can be found without sugar in it. I also use a lot of various types of herbs and spices to add different flavors to my food.

If I am very hungry, I will just double the portion sizes so that I feel full. Additionally, I have found many take out restaurants or fast food places where I can get flame broiled or grilled chicken and steamed vegetables or some variation of this. Also, many ethnic restaurants such as Greek, Middle Eastern, Asian, South American, Mexican, Cuban, African, Caribbean, Italian, Indian, etc., offer a variety of food choices consisting of meat, vegetables, and different types of bean dishes cooked in various ways. If I am not sure what is in the sauces, I just tell them to hold the sauce and they are fine. If for some reason, I am served a meal with a sauce on it that I am unfamiliar with,

I will just scrape off as much of it as I can. These places usually do not offer a sugar free salad dressing, so I just either eat the salad plain when I order a salad, or I will use a little olive oil or salsa, if available. As mentioned earlier though, I have found a sugar free salad dressing in the grocery markets. For the most part, I have not been hampered in any way whatsoever, from eating out at restaurants.

I will usually drink plain bottled water, water with a slice of lemon, herbal tea, or mineral water, with my lunch.

Afternoon Snack:

My afternoon snack usually consists of one of the following, with little variation, as I usually do not have a lot of time to devote towards thinking of something to eat.

- Nuts, which I eat until I feel I have had enough,

- Fish cups, like salmon or sometimes tuna,

- Boiled egg,

- Leftovers from lunch

Dinner:

Dinner is the same as lunch. I almost always make enough of dinner to take for my lunch the following day, so whatever is listed in lunch, is what I eat for dinner. I will also sometimes order take out or dine out as mentioned above. And, as you can see, there is still a wide variety of food options to indulge in and yet still stay within the dietary restrictions.

Other Meal Information:

In the summertime, when it is really hot out, I will sometimes make a pitcher of cold herb tea since there are many herb teas that give the illusion of being sweet because the flowers from which they are made have a strong, sweet smelling, aroma.

As for alcohol, I usually don't drink because the sugar in the alcohol can brings on symptoms. I will, from time to time, have a small glass of wine or a few sips of a margarita or something, when out for a nice dinner. But I always have food when drinking alcohol and do not drink alcohol on an empty stomach. Likewise, I try not to consume caffeinated tea or coffee, as caffeine stimulates the release of adrenalin, which in turn stimulates the release of sugar from the liver, which causes the pancreas to release too much insulin, which then drops the blood sugar level too low.

As far as holiday foods are concerned, I can usually find something to eat at parties so that I don't appear like I'm antisocial or something. Most holiday meals have some sort of meat that everything else is centered around, whether it be a turkey, a ham, or with summer holidays, barbecue meat of some sort.

The meats are usually safe to eat unless they have some sort of sauce on them, as in barbecue. I have not found any barbecue sauce on the market that doesn't have sugar in it. So, I will usually not eat barbecue meats unless I made it myself. In the summer, when I barbecue on the grill, I will use some kind of spicy hot sauce on the meat and it tastes delicious. In addition to the holiday meats, there are usually several side dishes to eat that are sugar free or are not a refined carbohydrate, such as various vegetable dishes. At Thanksgiving and Christmas, there are always the traditional vegetables served like squash, yams, string beans, spinach, salad, bean dishes, etc. to choose from. I avoid the dishes with potatoes, dressing, or noodles. Then there are the holiday desserts. I avoid all of them. And since I no longer crave sugar, it does not bother me if other people eat desserts in front of me. I have, however, learned how to make a sugar free pumpkin pie that is very good. You can find more information on how to make this in the chapter on Dessert Ideas.

When people at work see how often I eat, most all of them are shocked that I do not gain weight. To most of them, I eat a lot of food. But really, I probably eat the same amounts of food that other people do, mine are just spread out during the day, versus eating one or two large meals at one or two sittings. I've never really had a tendency to gain weight, although I probably could if I wanted to make an effort to do so. I am 5'4" and my weight normally stays between 120-125 pounds. I would really have a hard time overeating because I always eat until I feel full, and then I stop. Unlike when I was a child, I no longer feel well when I stuff myself beyond fullness. About a year before I developed reactive hypoglycemia, I had a hard time just maintaining my weight and would often eat large amounts of food just not to lose weight. I remember specifically telling my doctor that I thought something was wrong because a person should not have to eat massive amounts of food just to maintain their weight. The doctor never had any explanation for it and when I would tell him that I would eat two burgers and a package of donuts for dinner, they would just tell me that it was unhealthy and that I shouldn't eat like that. Later, my endocrinologist told me that because I had a problem with carbohydrate metabolism, I was not absorbing carbohydrates properly, which affected my ability to maintain my weight. He informed me that once I changed the way I ate, not only would my hypoglycemic symptoms stabilize, but I would not have any problems maintaining my weight, which has ultimately turned out to be true.

Also, when it comes to illness, unlike a lot of people who gets a cold, the flu, a toothache, or a stomachache, and just don't feel like eating, I have to force myself to eat because if I don't, I just feel worse from my blood sugar level being too low. Additionally, I have found many diabetic over the counter medicines that are sugar free that I will use when I am sick.

In the beginning, when my blood sugar was erratic, I used a blood sugar monitor to test my sugar every time I ate. I would test the first half hour after I ate, then again on the hour, then an hour later, and an hour after that. I wanted to see how different foods affected me. I would keep a notebook and record all my sugar levels, what I had eaten, and when I had eaten. During that time, there were many instances when I had blood sugar readings in the 50's. Sometimes I would wake up in the night or early in the morning with a reading in the 50's. Needless to say, I felt very sick during those times. Normal is approximately 80-100mg. I have never had a reading lower than 50 though. I can't imagine what that must feel like. Also, in the beginning, I never had a reading that went as high as 90-100mg. Now however, with the new way that I eat, I have had blood sugar readings into the 90's, which makes me feel good to see that because I know that not only do I feel great, but my body is stabilized. Now I rarely use my blood sugar monitor except if I am feeling unusually low for some unknown reason or if I am having lows for several days in a row for some reason, which for me now, is unusual.

NOTES

5

EXERCISE

EXERCISE

Exercise can be a double aged sword. While exercise helps counteract insulin resistance by making your cells more receptive to insulin, exercise lowers the blood sugar, in everybody, and in someone with reactive hypoglycemia who has not yet stabilized their blood sugar, exercise will cause the blood sugar to drop even lower and bring on symptoms. Furthermore, exercise has a carryover effect and will cause the blood sugar to stay lower even into the next day and sometimes, the next few days.

When I first developed reactive hypoglycemia, I had been getting regular exercise. In fact, the severity of my symptoms occurred shortly after I had participated in a 5K running event. During that time, I had no energy or was in the frame of mind to even think about exercising. However, as I began to get my blood sugar under control, I was slowly able to add exercise back into my lifestyle. Now that I eat correctly, I participate in many sporting events with no problems and have received numerous medals from competing in events including running, skating, and cycling.

My normal exercise routine involves working out approximately three times a week. When I am training for a 5K or other event, I will often work out four times a week. I usually run on the treadmill for about 30 minutes and then work out with the weight machines for about 30 minutes. Sometimes I will go running on the track at the local college or I will go on a bike ride or go skating instead.

During times when I slack off and don't exercise for several months, and then try to resume my regular workout routine, I will often start to have minor hypoglycemic reactions even though I am following a correct diet. During times like this, I usually have to adjust the times that I eat up by a half hour. So for example, instead of eating every three hours, I will eat every two and a half hours. After a few days, my body adjusts to the increased exercise and I am fine again. I am not sure why this happens, but maybe the body gets used to a certain energy level and when you increase it, it takes time to adjust.

When I am following my normal workout schedule though, it becomes very important to adhere to eating correctly and eating in intervals, as the glycogen reserves in your liver often gets used up from the exercise, and to restore this reserve, you have to take in enough carbohydrates to replenish it, as well as enough to keep your body fueled to function properly. Which is why after an extraordinary bout of strenuous or lengthy exercise, such as a marathon, it may take a few days to stabilize again, because you have no reserve sugar left to draw on from your liver during a low blood sugar attack since it was all used up during the intensive event.

Although I have never ran a marathon, I have participated in the Los Angeles bike tour, which is held the morning of the Los Angeles marathon, and consists of cycling for 26 miles, the length of a marathon. I have done this event several times, as well as participated in 26 mile bike tours in other cities. These types of lengthy events can be very challenging and requires that you maintain a stable blood sugar level throughout the event. Therefore, if you have not been eating properly leading up to the event and have been experiencing ups and downs in your blood sugar levels, it would probably not be wise to attempt this kind of event until you have stabilized. Additionally, I always ensure that I eat an adequate amount of food for several days after such an event to replenish the glycogen stores in the liver that will have been exhausted during such a race.

Also, at many of these athletic events, they often serve post race snacks, consisting primarily of sugary foods. I have participated in numerous of these events, and invariably, the post race snacks consist of fruit juices or sugary sports drinks, athletic bars high in sugar, bagels, which are made from refined flour, and various types of fruit. I rarely see any protein being offered or whole grain foods. Knowing what to expect, I will usually either bring my own snack, wait to eat when I get home, or stop somewhere and pick up something to eat on the way home.

NOTES

6

DESSERT IDEAS

DESSERT IDEAS

Just about any dessert recipe can be modified to make the dish sugar free and without refined carbohydrates. I rarely eat desserts, except occasionally during the holidays. The following are some desserts that I have made by modifying the recipes. They are tasty and do not include sugar, refined carbohydrates, dairy, fruit juice, or honey. However, even these desserts are only to be eaten occasionally because many with reactive hypoglycemia cannot tolerate to eat them more often.

PUMPKIN PIE

2 cans of sugar free pumpkins

Allspice

Cinnamon

Nutmeg

Almond flour

Chopped pecans

Olive oil

Butter or butter substitute

Mix the canned pumpkins, allspice, and nutmeg together in a bowl. I do not use a specific measurement for the spices, I just season it until it tastes the way I want it to taste. Then in another bowl, mix the almond flour, one half teaspoon of cinnamon, two tablespoons of butter and two tablespoons of olive oil. Press this into a lightly greased pie pan to form the piecrust. Pour in the pumpkin mixture. Sprinkle chopped pecans in the center. Bake at 375 degrees for 45 minutes. Let cool. Then enjoy.

FROZEN BERRY DELIGHT

One bag of mixed frozen berries
Crushed mixed nuts
Unsweetened flaked coconut
Unsweetened vanilla soymilk

Fill a tall clear glass one fourth of the way with the frozen berries. Then add a layer of the mixed nuts, and continue alternating berries and nuts until the glass is full. Sprinkle a handful of the unsweetened coconut flakes on top. Pour in one-fourth cup of cold, unsweetened, vanilla soymilk. Enjoy!

STRAWBERRY SMOOTHIE

Unsweetened vanilla soymilk
Almond flour
Frozen strawberries
Carbonated water
Crushed ice

Blend until smooth, a half cup of frozen strawberries, two tablespoons of almond flour, a half cup of unsweetened vanilla soymilk, one-fourth cup of carbonated water, and a handful of crushed ice. Serve.

BLUEBERRY MUFFINS

Almond flour
Baking powder
Egg
Olive Oil
Fresh blueberries
Unsweetened plain soymilk
Flaxseeds or sesame seeds
Chopped pecans or walnuts (optional)

Combine one cup of almond flour, one and one-fourth tea-
spoons of baking powder, one egg, one-fourth cup of soymilk,
a half cup of fresh blueberries, and two tablespoons of olive
oil, and mix until smooth. Add in a handful of chopped nuts if
desired. Lightly oil a six container muffin pan with olive oil.
Pour mixture into the muffin pan. Sprinkle flaxseeds or sesame seeds on top of each muffin. Bake at 400 degrees for 25 to
30 minutes. Let cool, then serve.

NOTES

7

HELPFUL HINTS AND TIPS

HELPFUL HINTS AND TIPS

- Purchase a blood sugar monitor

- Consider purchasing a medical alert bracelet if you have severe symptoms

- See an Endocrinologist instead of a general practitioner

- Read books and research online about reactive hypoglycemia and diabetes

- Join an online support group if you have no one to talk to and need a supportive ear

- Learn about diabetes mellitus, type II, as a lot of information also applies to reactive hypoglycemia

- Exercise

- Consider taking vitamins

- Cut down on your stress level as adrenalin causes the liver to release sugar in the form of gylcogen, which raises the blood sugar and causes the pancreas to release insulin to lower your blood sugar level

- Get a copy of the Glycemic index, which is a listing of foods and the speed in which these foods are metabolized in the body

- Consider buying a watch with an alarm that you can set to remind yourself when to eat if you are the type of person who skips meals

- Consider keeping some hard candy with you in case of an emergency

- Consider buying diabetic cough syrup and other diabetic products that are sugar free

NOTES

CONCLUSION

CONCLUSION

Reactive hypoglycemia is a condition that requires discipline and a change of eating habits if you want to experience good health. I am an example of how you can stabilize your blood sugar level and enjoy your life. Once you develop eating habits that work best for your body, reactive hypoglycemia does not have to interfere with your life or be a detriment to things you want to accomplish. For me, the key is discipline. That is the foundation of being able to live as a functional human being. And being disciplined comes by accepting the fact that you cannot eat like most other people do, or you will get sick, period. Learn to accept yourself for who you are and do what you have to do. Your body will reward you with abundant energy and good health. And you will find that all the severe, debilitating symptoms will stay away.

ABOUT THE AUTHOR

K. E. Lytle is a native Californian. K. E. Lytle is a graduate of California State University, Los Angeles, with a Bachelor's of Arts degree in Child Education. To contact K. E. Lytle, please write to:

> K. E. Lytle
> P.O. Box 241794
> Los Angeles, CA
> 90024

978-0-595-47021-1
0-595-47021-1